I0416764

OSTEOPOROSIS DIET COOKBOOK FOR SENIORS

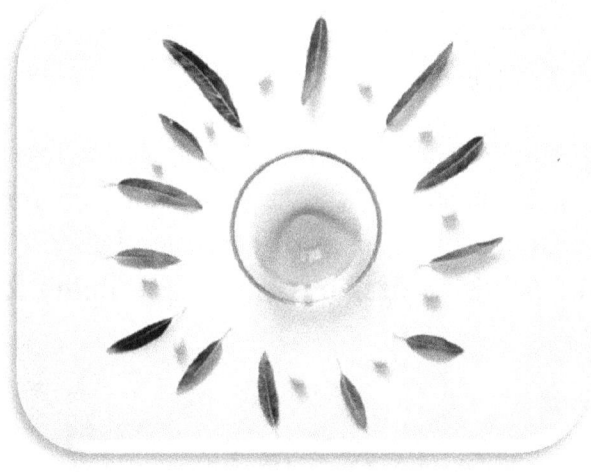

An ultimate Nutrition Guide for healthy bone and rich calcium for Seniors with Osteoporosis

Dr. Linda McDaniel

Text Copyright© 2024 by Dr. Linda McDaniel

All rights reserved worldwide No part of this publication may be republished in any form or by any means, including photocopying, scanning or otherwise without prior written permission to the copyright holder.

This book contains nonfictional content. The views expressed are those of the author and do not necessarily represent those of the publisher. In addition, the publisher declaims any responsibility for them.

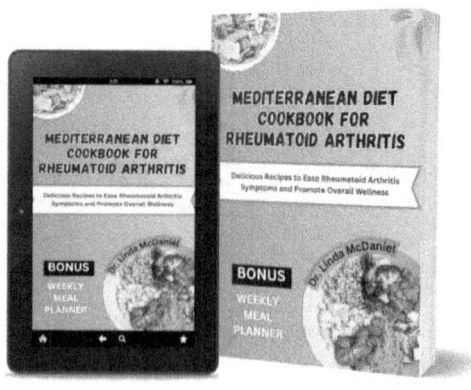

TABLE OF CONTENT

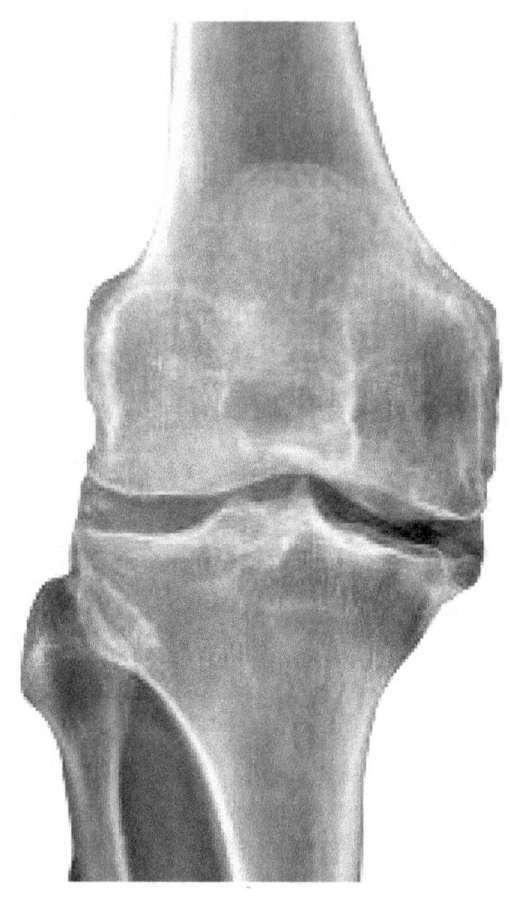

INTRODUCTION

Osteoporosis, a condition characterized by weakened bones and increased risk of fractures, is a significant health concern for seniors. As we age, our bones naturally lose density and strength, making us more susceptible to fractures from even minor falls or impacts. For seniors, particularly women post-menopause, osteoporosis poses a serious threat to quality of life, mobility, and independence.

Understanding the importance of diet in managing osteoporosis is paramount. A balanced and nutrient-rich diet can play a crucial role in maintaining bone health and even slowing the progression of osteoporosis. By focusing on foods that are rich in calcium, vitamin D, magnesium, and other essential nutrients, individuals can support bone density and strength.

Finding help with the right diet involves making informed choices about the foods we consume. This cookbook aims to provide seniors with a comprehensive guide to nutritious and delicious recipes specifically designed to combat osteoporosis. By incorporating anti-inflammatory ingredients and prioritizing bone-supportive nutrients, these recipes offer a practical and enjoyable way for individuals to take control of their bone health and enhance their overall well-being. Whether you're newly diagnosed with osteoporosis or seeking to manage its effects, this cookbook serves as a valuable resource on the journey to stronger bones and a healthier lifestyle.

CHAPTER 1:

Understanding Osteoporosis

Osteoporosis is a common bone disease characterized by decreased bone density and quality, leading to an increased risk of fractures. It affects millions of people worldwide, especially older adults, and can have significant impacts on mobility, independence, and overall quality of life. In this comprehensive guide, we will delve into the various aspects of osteoporosis, including its types, causes, symptoms, and preventive measures, to provide a deeper understanding of this condition and empower individuals to take proactive steps towards bone health.

Types of Osteoporosis

Primary and secondary osteoporosis are the two main forms of the disease. Primary osteoporosis is the most common form and typically occurs due to the natural aging process or hormonal changes, such as menopause in women and decreased testosterone levels in men. Secondary osteoporosis, on the other hand, is caused by underlying medical conditions or medications that affect bone health, such as long-term use of corticosteroids or certain chronic diseases like rheumatoid arthritis.

Causes of Osteoporosis

The development of osteoporosis is influenced by various factors, including genetics, lifestyle choices, and medical history. One of the main contributors to osteoporosis is a decrease in bone density over time, which can occur due to age-related hormonal changes, inadequate nutrition, or sedentary lifestyle. Other risk factors include a family history of osteoporosis, certain medical conditions like thyroid disorders or gastrointestinal diseases, and lifestyle habits such as smoking, excessive alcohol consumption, and lack of exercise.

Symptoms of Osteoporosis

Osteoporosis is commonly known as a "silent disease" since it usually worsens without causing any symptoms until a fracture. However, as bone density decreases, individuals may experience symptoms such as back pain, loss of height, stooped posture, and fractures that occur with minimal trauma or pressure. Fractures commonly occur in the spine, hip, and wrist and can significantly impact mobility and daily activities.

Preventive Measures for Osteoporosis: While osteoporosis cannot always be prevented, there are several proactive measures individuals can take to reduce their risk and maintain bone health.

These include:

1. **Adequate Calcium and Vitamin D Intake:** Calcium is essential for bone health, and vitamin D helps the body absorb calcium effectively. Consuming foods rich in calcium, such as dairy products, leafy greens, and fortified foods, and getting plenty of sunlight exposure or taking vitamin D supplements can support bone density.

2. **Regular Exercise:** Weight-bearing and resistance exercises, such as walking, jogging, strength training, and yoga, help strengthen bones and improve balance and coordination, reducing the risk of falls and fractures.

3. **Healthy Lifestyle Choices:** Avoiding smoking, limiting alcohol consumption, and maintaining a healthy body weight can all contribute to better bone health and overall well-being.

4. **Bone Density Testing:** Regular bone density scans, such as dual-energy X-ray absorptiometry (DXA) scans, can help monitor bone health and detect osteoporosis early, allowing for timely intervention and treatment.

5. **Medication and Treatment:** In some cases, healthcare providers may prescribe medications, such as bisphosphonates or hormone therapy, to help slow the progression of osteoporosis and reduce the risk of fractures.

Osteoporosis is a significant health concern affecting millions of individuals worldwide, particularly older adults. By understanding the types, causes, symptoms, and preventive measures associated with osteoporosis, individuals can take proactive steps to protect their bone health and reduce their risk of fractures. Through a combination of healthy lifestyle choices, adequate nutrition, regular exercise, and medical intervention when necessary, it is possible to maintain strong and healthy bones throughout life, promoting overall well-being and quality of life.

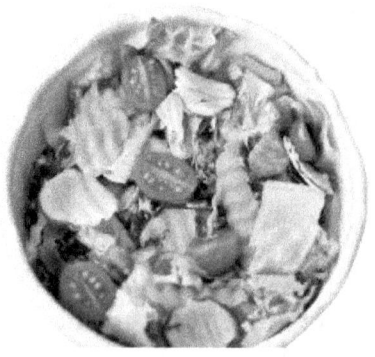

Chapter 2:

DIETARY CHOICES

Achieving optimum health with osteoporosis involves making informed dietary choices that support bone density, reduce inflammation, and promote overall well-being. Here's a guide to the foods to eat and avoid for an osteoporosis diet:

Foods to Eat:

1. **Calcium-Rich Foods:** Calcium is essential for maintaining strong bones and preventing osteoporosis. Incorporate calcium-rich foods into your diet, such as dairy products like milk, cheese, and yogurt, as well as fortified foods like tofu, orange juice, and cereals.

2. **Leafy Greens:** Dark, leafy greens like kale, spinach, collard greens, and Swiss chard are excellent sources of calcium, as well as other bone-supporting nutrients like vitamin K and magnesium.

3. **Salmon and Other Fatty Fish:** Fatty fish like salmon, sardines, and mackerel are rich in omega-3 fatty acids,

which have anti-inflammatory properties and can help reduce the risk of osteoporosis-related fractures.

4. Nuts and Seeds: Almonds, walnuts, sesame seeds, and chia seeds are packed with calcium, magnesium, and other nutrients that support bone health. They also provide healthy fats and protein for overall wellness.

5. Fortified Foods: Incorporate fortified foods into your diet, such as fortified plant-based milk alternatives (e.g., almond milk, soy milk), fortified cereals, and fortified tofu, to increase your intake of calcium and vitamin D.

6. Fruits and Vegetables: Aim to include a variety of fruits and vegetables in your diet, as they provide essential vitamins, minerals, and antioxidants that support overall health and may help reduce inflammation.

Foods to Avoid or Limit:

1. Excessive Sodium: High sodium intake can lead to calcium loss in the bones and increase the risk of osteoporosis. Limit your consumption of processed foods, canned soups,

salty snacks, and fast food, and opt for low-sodium alternatives whenever possible.

2. Caffeine: While moderate caffeine consumption is generally safe, excessive intake may interfere with calcium absorption and increase the risk of bone loss. Limit your intake of caffeinated beverages like coffee, tea, and soda, and opt for decaffeinated versions or alternative drinks like herbal tea or water.

3. Alcohol: Heavy alcohol consumption can negatively impact bone health by interfering with calcium absorption and increasing the risk of falls and fractures. Limit your alcohol intake to no more than one drink per day for women and two drinks per day for men, and consider avoiding alcohol altogether if you have osteoporosis or are at risk of fractures.

4. High Acidic Foods: Foods that are high in acid, such as processed meats, refined grains, and sugary snacks, may contribute to inflammation and bone loss. Limit your intake of these foods and focus on consuming a balanced diet rich in whole, nutrient-dense foods instead.

5. **Carbonated Beverages:** Soda and other carbonated beverages contain phosphoric acid, which may leach calcium from the bones and increase the risk of osteoporosis. Opt for water, herbal tea, or calcium-fortified beverages as healthier alternatives.

By incorporating these dietary guidelines into your daily routine, you can support bone health, reduce inflammation, and promote overall wellness while managing osteoporosis effectively.

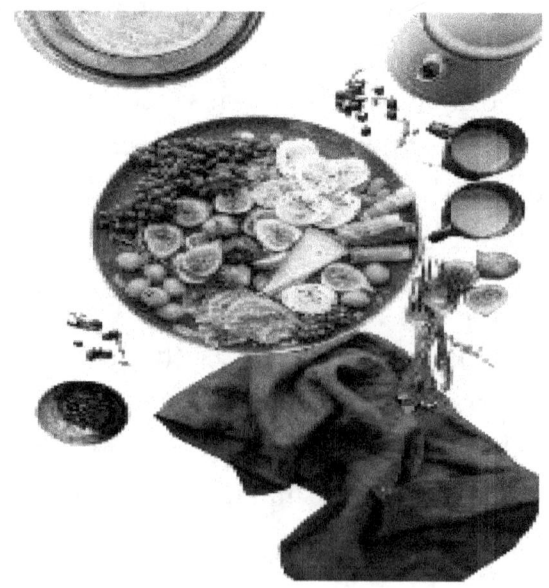

CHAPTER 3:

DIETERY PLAN

Following an osteoporosis diet for seniors involves making strategic dietary choices to support bone health, reduce inflammation, and maintain overall well-being. Here's a step-by-step guide on how seniors can effectively follow an osteoporosis diet:

1. Consult with a Healthcare Professional: Before making any significant changes to your diet, it's essential to consult with your healthcare provider or a registered dietitian. They can assess your individual nutritional needs, medical history, and any specific dietary restrictions or considerations related to osteoporosis.

2. Educate Yourself: Take the time to learn about the principles of an osteoporosis diet and understand which foods are beneficial for bone health and which ones to avoid or limit. Knowledge is empowering and will help you make informed decisions about your dietary choices.

3. **Plan Balanced Meals:** Aim to include a variety of nutrient-rich foods in your meals to ensure you're getting all the essential vitamins, minerals, and antioxidants needed for bone health. Focus on incorporating calcium-rich foods, such as dairy products, leafy greens, fortified foods, and protein sources like lean meats, fish, eggs, tofu, and legumes.

4. **Emphasize Calcium and Vitamin D:** Calcium and vitamin D are crucial nutrients for maintaining strong bones. Ensure you're meeting your daily recommended intake of calcium (1,000-1,200 mg/day for adults over 50) and vitamin D (600-800 IU/day for adults over 50) through a combination of dietary sources and supplements, if necessary.

5. **Include Anti-Inflammatory Foods:** Chronic inflammation can contribute to bone loss and increase the risk of fractures. Incorporate anti-inflammatory foods into your diet, such as fatty fish rich in omega-3 fatty acids, fruits, vegetables, nuts, seeds, and whole grains.

6. **Limit Sodium and Acidic Foods:** Excessive sodium intake can lead to calcium loss in the bones, while acidic foods may contribute to inflammation and bone loss. Limit your consumption of high-sodium processed foods, salty snacks,

and acidic foods like processed meats, refined grains, sugary snacks, and carbonated beverages.

7. Stay Hydrated: Adequate hydration is essential for overall health and can help maintain bone density. Aim to drink plenty of water throughout the day and limit your intake of caffeinated and alcoholic beverages, which can have a diuretic effect and contribute to dehydration.

8. Monitor Portion Sizes: Pay attention to portion sizes to avoid overeating, which can lead to weight gain and put extra stress on your bones. Practice mindful eating and listen to your body's hunger and fullness cues to maintain a healthy weight and support bone health.

9. Be Consistent: Consistency is key when following an osteoporosis diet. Aim to make healthy dietary choices consistently over time, rather than relying on occasional or sporadic changes. Remember that small, sustainable changes can lead to significant improvements in bone health and overall well-being.

10. Reevaluate and Adjust: Regularly reassess your dietary habits and make adjustments as needed based on your health goals, lifestyle changes, and any new recommendations from your healthcare provider or dietitian.

Flexibility and adaptability are essential for long-term success in maintaining an osteoporosis-friendly diet.

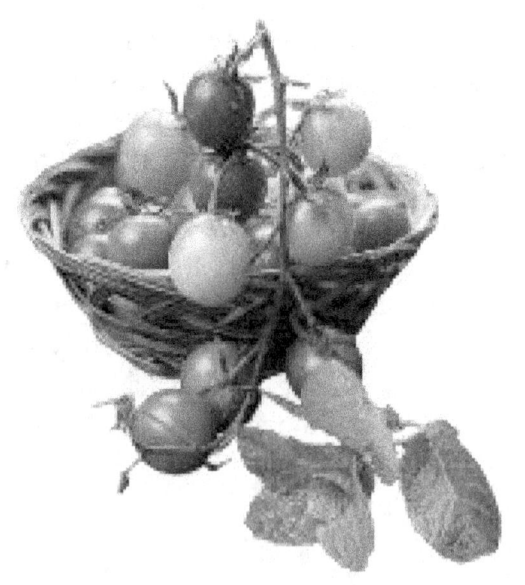

CHAPTER 4:

Breakfast:

❖ **Calcium-Rich Yogurt Parfait:**

Ingredients:

- 1 cup low-fat Greek yogurt
- 1/2 cup fresh berries (such as strawberries, blueberries, or raspberries)
- 2 tablespoons chopped almonds or walnuts, 1 tablespoon honey or maple syrup

Preparation:

1. In a bowl or glass, layer the Greek yogurt, fresh berries, and chopped nuts.

2. Drizzle honey or maple syrup on top for added sweetness.

3. Serve immediately and enjoy!

Cooking Time: 5 minutes

Nutritional Value: Calories: 250 calories, Protein: 20 grams, Calcium: 300 milligrams, Fiber: 5 grams

❖ **Spinach and Feta Omelette:**

Ingredients:

- 2 large egg, 1/2 cup fresh spinach leaves, 1/4 cup crumbled feta cheese, Salt and pepper to taste, 1 teaspoon olive oil

Preparation:

1. Beat the eggs in a bowl until thoroughly blended. Season with salt and pepper.

2. Heat olive oil in a non-stick skillet over medium heat. when the spinach has wilted, add the leaves and simmer. .

3. Pour the beaten eggs into the skillet, swirling to evenly distribute.

4. Sprinkle the crumbled feta cheese over one half of the omelette.

5. Once the eggs are set, fold the omelette in half and cook for another minute or until the cheese is melted then transfer to a plate and serve hot.

Cooking Time: 10 minutes

Nutritional Value: Calories: 250 calories, Protein: 20 grams, Calcium: 150 milligrams, Fiber: 2 grams

❖ Overnight Oats with Chia Seeds:

Ingredients:

- 1/2 cup rolled oats, 1/2 cup low-fat milk or almond milk
- 1 tablespoon chia seeds, 1/2 teaspoon vanilla extract, 1 tablespoon honey or maple syrup
- 1/4 cup sliced bananas or berries (optional)

Preparation:

1. In a jar or bowl, combine the rolled oats, milk, chia seeds, vanilla extract, and honey or maple syrup. Stir well to combine.

2. Cover and refrigerate overnight, or for at least 4 hours, to allow the oats to soften and absorb the liquid.

3. Before serving, stir in sliced bananas or berries if desired.

4. Enjoy cold or heat in the microwave for 1-2 minutes until warm.

Cooking Time: 5 minutes (plus overnight soaking)

Nutritional Value: Calories: 300 calories

Protein: 10 grams, Calcium: 150 milligrams, Fiber: 7 grams

❖ **Quinoa Breakfast Bowl with Almond Butter and Fruit:**

Ingredients:

- 1/2 cup cooked quinoa, 2 tablespoons almond butter
- 1/4 cup sliced bananas or berries
- 1 tablespoon chopped nuts or seeds (such as almonds, walnuts, or chia seeds)
- 1 teaspoon honey or maple syrup

Preparation:

1. In a bowl, combine the cooked quinoa and almond butter, stirring until well mixed.

2. Top the quinoa with sliced bananas or berries, chopped nuts or seeds, and a drizzle of honey or maple syrup.

3. . Gently stir to mix all the ingredients together.

4. Serve warm or at room temperature.

Cooking Time: 10 minutes (plus cooking quinoa)

Nutritional Value: Calories: 350 calories, Protein: 12 grams, Calcium: 50 milligrams, Fiber: 6 grams

❖ Greek Yogurt Smoothie with Kale and Pineapple:

Ingredients: 1/2 cup low-fat Greek yogurt, 1/2 cup unsweetened almond milk

- 1 cup fresh kale leaves, stems removed, 1/2 cup frozen pineapple chunks, 1 tablespoon chia seeds
- 1 teaspoon honey or maple syrup (optional)

Preparation:

1. In a blender, combine the Greek yogurt, almond milk, kale leaves, frozen pineapple chunks, and chia seeds.

2. Blend until smooth and creamy, adding more almond milk if needed to reach your desired consistency.

3. Taste and sweeten with honey or maple syrup if desired.

4. .Pour the smoothie into a glass and serve immediately.

Cooking Time: 5 minutes

Nutritional Value: Calories: 250 calories Protein: 15 grams, Calcium: 250 milligrams, Fiber: 8 grams

❖ Chia Seed Pudding with Berries and Almonds:

Ingredients:

- 1 tablespoon honey or maple 1/4 cup chia seeds, 1/2 teaspoon vanilla essence, and 1 cup unsweetened almond milk syrup, 1/4 cup mixed berries (such as strawberries, blueberries, or raspberries), 1 tablespoon chopped almonds

Preparation:

1. In a jar or bowl, combine the chia seeds, almond milk, vanilla extract, and honey or maple syrup. Stir well to combine.

2. Cover and refrigerate for at least 2 hours, or overnight, to allow the chia seeds to absorb the liquid and thicken.

3. Before serving, stir the chia seed pudding to redistribute the seeds evenly.

4. Top with mixed berries and chopped almonds.

5. Serve chilled.

Cooking Time: 5 minutes (plus chilling time)

Nutritional Value: Calories: 300 calories, Protein: 10 grams, Calcium: 250 milligrams, Fiber: 12 grams

Lunch:

❖ **Grilled Salmon Salad:**

Ingredients:

- 4 oz grilled salmon fillet, 2 cups mixed salad greens (such as spinach, arugula, and romaine), 1/4 cup cherry tomatoes, halved, 1/4 cup cucumber, sliced, 1/4 avocado, diced, 1 tablespoon olive oil, 1 tablespoon balsamic vinegar, Salt and pepper to taste

Preparation:

1. Season the salmon fillet with salt and pepper, then grill until cooked through.

2. In a large bowl, toss together the mixed salad greens, cherry tomatoes, cucumber, and avocado.

3. Drizzle with olive oil and balsamic vinegar, then toss to coat, top the salad with the grilled salmon, serve immediately.

Cooking Time: 15 minutes

Nutritional Value: Calories: 350 calories, Protein: 25 grams, Calcium: 100 milligrams, Fiber: 5 grams

❖ Quinoa and Vegetable Stir-Fry:

Ingredients:

- 1/2 cup cooked quinoa, 1/2 cup mixed vegetables (such as bell peppers, broccoli, carrots, and snap peas), 2 tablespoons low-sodium soy sauce, 1 tablespoon olive oil, 1 clove garlic, minced, 1/2 teaspoon grated ginger, Sesame seeds for garnish (optional)

Preparation:

1. Heat olive oil in a skillet or wok over medium-high heat.

2. Add the grated ginger and minced garlic, and cook for one to two minutes, or until fragrant.

3. Add mixed vegetables to the skillet and stir-fry until tender-crisp.

4. Stir in cooked quinoa and soy sauce, tossing to combine.

5. Cook for another 2-3 minutes until heated through. garnish with sesame seeds if desired.

Cooking Time: 15 minutes

Nutritional Value: Calories: 300 calories, Protein: 10 grams, Calcium: 50 milligrams, Fiber: 6 grams

❖ Lentil and Vegetable Soup:

Ingredients: 1/2 cup dried lentils, rinsed and drained, 2 cups low-sodium vegetable broth, 1 cup diced tomatoes

- 1/2 cup diced carrots, 1/2 cup diced celery, 1/2 cup diced onion, 1 clove garlic, minced, 1/2 teaspoon dried thyme, Salt and pepper to taste, Fresh parsley for garnish (optional)

Preparation:

1. In a large pot, combine lentils, vegetable broth, diced tomatoes, carrots, celery, onion, garlic, and thyme.

2. Bring to a boil over medium-high heat, then reduce heat to low and simmer for 20-25 minutes, or until lentils and vegetables are tender.

3. Season with salt and pepper to taste.

4. Ladle the soup into bowls and garnish with fresh parsley if desired then serve hot.

Cooking Time: 30 minutes

Nutritional Value: Calories: 250 calories, Protein: 15 grams, Calcium: 50 milligrams, Fiber: 10 grams

❖ Turkey and Vegetable Wrap:

Ingredients:

- 1 whole grain tortilla, 2 oz sliced turkey breast, 1/4 cup shredded lettuce, 1/4 cup sliced cucumber, 1/4 cup diced tomatoes
- One tablespoon each of hummus and Dijon mustard

Preparation:

1. Lay the whole grain tortilla flat on a clean surface.

2. Spread hummus evenly over the tortilla, leaving a small border around the edges.

3. Layer sliced turkey breast, shredded lettuce, sliced cucumber, and diced tomatoes on top of the hummus.

4. Drizzle with Dijon mustard.

5. Roll up the tortilla tightly to form a wrap.

6. Slice in half diagonally and serve immediately.

Cooking Time: 5 minutes

Nutritional Value: Calories: 300 calories, Protein: 20 grams, Calcium: 100 milligrams, Fiber:

❖ Chickpea and Vegetable Salad:

Ingredients:

- 1 cup canned chickpeas, rinsed and drained, 1/2 cup diced cucumber, 1/2 cup diced bell peppers (any color)

- 1/4 cup diced red onion, 2 tablespoons chopped fresh parsley, 1 tablespoon olive oil, 1 tablespoon lemon juice, Salt and pepper to taste

Preparation:

1. In a large bowl, combine chickpeas, diced cucumber, diced bell peppers, diced red onion, and chopped fresh parsley.

2. Drizzle with olive oil and lemon juice, then season with salt and pepper to taste.

3. Toss to coat all the ingredients evenly.

4. Serve chilled or at room temperature.

Cooking Time: 10 minutes

Nutritional Value: Calories: 250 calories, Protein: 10 grams, Calcium: 50 milligrams Fiber: 10 grams

❖ **Veggie and Hummus Wrap:**

Ingredients:

- 1 whole grain tortilla, 2 tablespoons hummus, 1/4 cup shredded carrots, 1/4 cup shredded lettuce, 1/4 cup sliced cucumber,1/4 cup sliced bell peppers (any color)

Preparation:

1. Lay the whole grain tortilla flat on a clean surface.

2. Spread hummus evenly over the tortilla, leaving a small border around the edges.

3. Layer shredded carrots, shredded lettuce, sliced cucumber, and sliced bell peppers on top of the hummus.

4. Roll up the tortilla tightly to form a wrap.

5. Slice in half diagonally and serve immediately.

Cooking Time: 5 minutes

Nutritional Value: Calories: 200 calories, Protein: 5 grams, Calcium: 50 milligrams, Fiber: 5 grams

❖ Greek Salad with Grilled Chicken:

Ingredients:

- 2 cups mixed salad greens (such as spinach, arugula, and romaine), 4 oz grilled chicken breast, sliced, 1/4 cup cherry tomatoes, halved, 1/4 cup diced cucumber

- 1/4 cup sliced black olives, 1/4 cup crumbled feta cheese, 1 tablespoon olive oil, 1 tablespoon red wine vinegar, Salt and pepper to taste

Preparation:

1. In a large bowl, combine mixed salad greens, sliced grilled chicken breast, cherry tomatoes, diced cucumber, sliced black olives, and crumbled feta cheese.

2. Drizzle with olive oil and red wine vinegar, then season with salt and pepper to taste.

3. Toss to coat all the ingredients evenly.

4. Serve immediately.

Cooking Time: 15 minutes

Nutritional Value: Calories: 350 calories Protein:30 grams, Calcium: 150 milligrams, Fiber: 5 grams

❖ **Tuna Salad Stuffed Avocado:**

Ingredients:

- 1 ripe avocado, 1/2 cup canned tuna, drained, 1/4 cup diced celery, 1/4 cup diced red onion, 1 tablespoon Greek yogurt, 1 teaspoon Dijon mustard, Salt and pepper to taste, Fresh parsley for garnish (optional)

Preparation:

1. Halve the ripe avocado and scoop out the pit.

2. In a bowl, combine canned tuna, diced celery, diced red onion, Greek yogurt, and Dijon mustard.

3. Season with salt and pepper to taste, then mix well to combine.

4. Spoon the tuna salad mixture into the avocado halves.

5. Garnish with fresh parsley if desired and serve immediately.

Cooking Time: 10 minutes

Nutritional Value: Calories: 300 calories, Protein: 20 grams, Calcium: 50 milligrams, Fiber: 5 grams

Dinner:

❖ **Baked Salmon with Roasted Vegetables:**

Ingredients: 4 oz salmon fillet, 1 cup mixed vegetables (such as broccoli, carrots, and bell peppers), chopped, 1 tablespoon olive oil, 1/2 teaspoon garlic powder, 1/2 teaspoon dried herbs (such as thyme or rosemary), Salt and pepper to taste

Preparation:

1. Preheat the oven to 400°F (200°C), place the salmon fillet on a baking sheet lined with parchment paper.

2. In a bowl, toss the mixed vegetables with olive oil, garlic powder, dried herbs, salt, and pepper.

3. Spread the seasoned vegetables around the salmon on the baking sheet.

4. Bake in the preheated oven for 15-20 minutes, or until the salmon is cooked through and the vegetables are tender and serve hot.

Cooking Time: 20 minutes

Nutritional Value: Calories: 300 calories, Protein: 25 grams, Calcium: 100 milligrams, Fiber: 5 grams

❖ Chicken and Vegetable Stir-Fry:

Ingredients: 4 oz boneless, skinless chicken breast, thinly sliced, 1 cup mixed vegetables (such as bell peppers, broccoli, and snap peas), sliced, 1 tablespoon low-sodium soy sauce, 1 tablespoon olive oil, 1 clove garlic, minced, 1/2 teaspoon grated ginger, Sesame seeds for garnish (optional)

Preparation:

1. Heat olive oil in a skillet or wok over medium-high heat, add minced garlic and grated ginger, and sauté for 1-2 minutes until fragrant.

2. Add sliced chicken breast to the skillet and stir-fry until cooked through.

3. Add mixed vegetables to the skillet and stir-fry until tender-crisp, stir in low-sodium soy sauce, tossing to combine.

4. Cook for another 2-3 minutes until heated through, garnish with sesame seeds if desired and serve hot.

Cooking Time: 15 minutes

Nutritional Value: Calories: 300 calories, Protein: 25 grams, Calcium: 100 milligrams, Fiber: 5 grams

❖ **Lentil Soup with Spinach:**

Ingredients:

- 1/2 cup dried green lentils, rinsed and drained

- 2 cups low-sodium vegetable broth, 1 cup diced tomatoes, 1 cup chopped spinach leaves, 1/2 cup diced onion, 1 clove garlic, minced, 1/2 teaspoon dried thyme, Salt and pepper to taste, Fresh parsley for garnish (optional)

Preparation:

1. In a large pot, combine dried green lentils, vegetable broth, diced tomatoes, chopped spinach leaves, diced onion, minced garlic, dried thyme, salt, and pepper.

2. Bring to a boil over medium-high heat, then reduce heat to low and simmer for 25-30 minutes, or until the lentils are tender.

3. Season with additional salt and pepper to taste.

4. Ladle the soup into bowls and garnish with fresh parsley if desired and serve hot.

Cooking Time: 35 minutes

Nutritional Value: Calories: 250 calories Protein: 15 grams, Calcium: y 50 milligrams, Fiber: 10 grams

Whole Grain Pasta Primavera:

Ingredients: 1 cup whole grain pasta, 1 cup mixed vegetables (such as bell peppers, zucchini, and cherry tomatoes), sliced, 2 tablespoons olive oil,1 clove garlic, minced, 1/4 teaspoon red pepper flakes (optional), Salt and pepper to taste, Grated Parmesan cheese for garnish (optional)

Preparation:

1. Cook the whole grain pasta according to package instructions until al dente. Drain and set aside, heat olive oil in a skillet over medium heat, add minced garlic and red pepper flakes (if using), and sauté for 1-2 minutes until fragrant.

2. Add mixed vegetables to the skillet and stir-fry until tender-crisp, season with salt and pepper to taste, add cooked pasta to the skillet and toss to combine.

3. Cook for another 2-3 minutes until heated through, serve hot, garnished with grated Parmesan cheese if desired.

Cooking Time: 20 minutes

Nutritional Value: Calories: 350 calories, Protein: 10 grams, Calcium: 50 milligrams, Fiber: 8 grams

❖ Turkey and Vegetable Skewers:

Ingredients: 4 oz turkey breast, cut into chunks, 1 cup mixed vegetables (such as bell peppers, onions, and mushrooms), cut into chunks, 1 tablespoon olive oil, 1 teaspoon Italian seasoning, Salt and pepper to taste

Preparation:

1. Preheat the grill or grill pan over medium-high heat, in a bowl, toss together turkey breast chunks, mixed vegetables, olive oil, Italian seasoning, salt, and pepper until well coated.

2. Thread the turkey and vegetable chunks onto skewers, alternating between turkey and vegetables.

3. Grill the skewers for 8-10 minutes, turning occasionally, until the turkey is cooked through and the vegetables are tender, remove from the grill and serve hot.

Cooking Time: 15 minutes

Nutritional Value: Calories 250 calories, Protein: 25 grams, Calcium: 100 milligrams, Fiber: 5 grams

❖ Bean and Vegetable Chili:

Ingredients: 1 can (15 oz) mixed beans (such as kidney beans, black beans, and cannellini beans), rinsed and drained, 1 cup diced tomatoes, 1/2 cup diced bell peppers (any color), 1/2 cup diced onion, 1 clove garlic, minced, 1 tablespoon olive oil, 1 teaspoon chili powder, 1/2 teaspoon cumin, Salt and pepper to taste, Fresh cilantro for garnish (optional)

Preparation:

1. Heat olive oil in a large pot over medium heat, add minced garlic, diced onion, and diced bell peppers to the pot, and sauté for 3-4 minutes until softened, stir in diced tomatoes, mixed beans, chili powder, cumin, salt, and pepper.

2. Bring the chili to a simmer, then reduce heat to low and cook for 20-25 minutes, stirring occasionally, until flavors are well blended.

3. Taste and adjust seasoning if needed, Ladle the chili into bowls and garnish with fresh cilantro if desired and serve hot.

Cooking Time: 30 minutes

Nutritional Value: Calories: 300 calories, Protein: 15 grams, Calcium: 100 milligrams, Fiber: 10 grams

Dessert:

❖ **Berry Yogurt Parfait Mixed :**

Ingredients:

- 1/2 cup low-fat Greek yogurt, 1/4 cup mixed berries (such as strawberries, blueberries, and raspberries),

- 1 tablespoon honey or maple syrup

- 2 tablespoons granola

Preparation:

1. In a glass or bowl, layer low-fat Greek yogurt, mixed berries, and honey or maple syrup.

2. Top with granola for added crunch.

3. Repeat the layers if desired,

4. serve immediately.

Preparation Time: 5 minutes

Nutritional Value: Calories: 150 calories, Protein: 8 grams, Calcium: 150 milligrams, Fiber: 3 grams

❖ Baked Apple with Cinnamon:

Ingredients:

- 1 medium apple, cored, 1 teaspoon cinnamon, 1 teaspoon honey or maple syrup,1 tablespoon chopped walnuts (optional)

Preparation:

1. Preheat the oven to 375°F (190°C).

2. Place the cored apple in a baking dish.

3. Sprinkle cinnamon over the apple and drizzle with honey or maple syrup.

4. Optionally, sprinkle chopped walnuts over the top.

5. Bake in the preheated oven for 20-25 minutes, or until the apple is tender.

6. Serve warm.

Cooking Time: 25 minutes

Nutritional Value: Calories: 100 calories, Protein: 1 gram, Calcium: 10 milligrams, Fiber: 4 grams

❖ Banana and Peanut Butter Bites:

Ingredients:

- 1 medium banana, sliced
- 2 tablespoons natural peanut butter
- 1 tablespoon dark chocolate chips (optional)
Preparation:

1. Spread natural peanut butter on banana slices.

2. Optionally, top each banana slice with a dark chocolate chip.

3. Serve immediately.

Preparation Time: 5 minutes

Nutritional Value:

Calories: 150 calories

Protein: y 4 grams

Calcium: 10 milligrams

Fiber: 3 grams

❖ **Honey and Almonds with Greek Yogourt:**

Ingredients:

- 1/2 cup low-fat Greek yogurt

- 1 tablespoon honey

- 1 tablespoon chopped almonds Preparation:

1. In a bowl, combine low-fat Greek yogurt and honey.

2. Top with chopped almonds.

3. Serve chilled.

Preparation Time: 5 minutes

Nutritional Value:

Calories: 150 calories

Protein: 10 grams

Calcium: 150 milligrams

Fiber: 1 gram

❖ Cottage Cheese with Pineapple:

Ingredients:

- 1/2 cup low-fat cottage cheese
- 1/4 cup diced pineapple
- 1 tablespoon shredded coconut (optional)
Preparation:

1. In a bowl, combine low-fat cottage cheese and diced pineapple.

2. Optionally, sprinkle shredded coconut over the top.

3. Serve chilled.

Preparation Time: 5 minutes

Nutritional Value:

Calories: 100 calories

Protein: 15 grams

Calcium: 100 milligrams

Fiber: 1 gram

❖ Frozen Banana Pops:

Ingredients:

- 1 ripe banana, peeled and cut into chunks, 1/4 cup dark chocolate chips, 1 tablespoon chopped nuts (such as almonds or peanuts), Wooden popsicle sticks

Preparation:

1. Insert a wooden popsicle stick into each banana chunk, place the banana pops on a baking sheet lined with parchment paper.

2. Melt dark chocolate chips in the microwave or over a double boiler.

3. Dip each banana pop into the melted chocolate, then sprinkle chopped nuts over the chocolate.

4. Place the banana pops in the freezer for at least 1 hour, or until the chocolate is set, serve frozen.

Preparation Time: 10 minutes (plus freezing time)

Nutritional Value: Calories: 100 calories, Protein: 2 grams, Calcium: 10 milligrams, Fiber: 2 grams

❖ **Berry Smoothie:**

Ingredients:

- Half a cup of mixed berries, including blueberries, raspberries, and strawberries

- 1/2 cup low-fat yogurt (any flavor)

- 1/2 cup almond milk

- 1 tablespoon honey or maple syrup (optional)
Preparation:

1. In a blender, combine mixed berries, low-fat yogurt, almond milk, and honey or maple syrup if desired.

2. Blend until smooth and creamy.

3. Pour into glasses and serve immediately.

Preparation Time: 5 minutes

Nutritional Value: Calories: 150 calories, Protein: 5 grams, Calcium: 150 milligrams, Fiber: 3 grams

❖ Pumpkin Chia Seed Pudding:

Ingredients:

- 1/4 cup canned pumpkin puree

- 1/2 cup almond milk, 2 tablespoons chia seeds

- 1 tablespoon maple syrup, 1/2 teaspoon pumpkin pie spice

Preparation:

1. In a jar or bowl, combine canned pumpkin puree, almond milk, chia seeds, maple syrup, and pumpkin pie spice, stir well to combine.

2. Cover and refrigerate for at least 2 hours, or overnight, to allow the chia seeds to absorb the liquid and thicken.

3. Stir the chia seed pudding before serving then serve chilled.

Preparation Time: 5 minutes (plus chilling time)

Nutritional Value: Calories: 150 calories, Protein: 5 grams, Calcium: 150 milligrams Fiber: 10 grams

❖ Almond Butter Stuffed Dates:

Ingredients:

- 4 large Medjool dates, pitted

- 2 tablespoons almond butter

- 1 tablespoon shredded coconut (optional)
Preparation:

1. Slice each Medjool date lengthwise, being careful not to cut all the way through.

2. Fill each date with almond butter.

3. Optionally, sprinkle shredded coconut over the top.

4. Serve immediately.

Preparation Time: 5 minutes

Nutritional Value: Calories: 150 calories, Protein: 3 grams, Calcium: 30 milligrams, Fiber: 4 grams

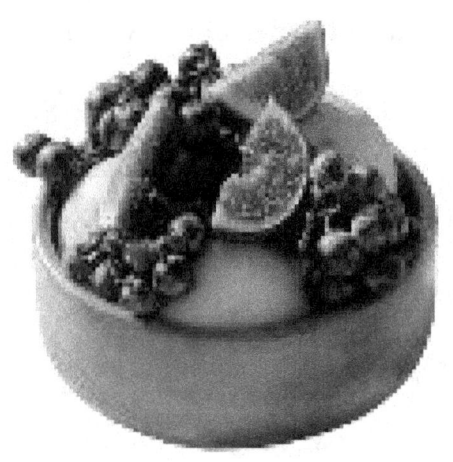

CONCLUSION

In conclusion, this Osteoporosis for Seniors cookbook serves as a valuable resource for individuals seeking to enhance their bone health and overall well-being through nutritious and delicious meals. Throughout the recipes provided, emphasis has been placed on incorporating ingredients rich in calcium, vitamin D, protein, and other essential nutrients known to support bone density and strength. From breakfast to dinner, and even dessert, these recipes offer a diverse range of options to suit various tastes and dietary preferences.

By following the guidelines outlined in this cookbook, seniors can proactively manage osteoporosis and reduce their risk of fractures and other complications associated with bone loss. The inclusion of nutrient-dense foods such as leafy greens, dairy products, lean proteins, whole grains, and fruits ensures that individuals receive the necessary nutrients to maintain optimal bone health.

Moreover, the simplicity of the recipes and the accessibility of the ingredients make it easier for seniors to incorporate these meals into their daily routine. Whether cooking for oneself or for loved ones, these recipes prioritize convenience without compromising on flavor or nutritional value.

As readers embark on their journey to adopt and adapt to this osteoporosis-friendly diet, it is essential to remember the profound impact that dietary choices can have on overall health and quality of life. By embracing this cookbook and committing to a balanced and nourishing diet, individuals can take proactive steps towards preserving bone health and enjoying a vibrant and active lifestyle well into their golden years.

In the words of Benjamin Franklin, "An ounce of prevention is worth a pound of cure." Therefore, let this cookbook serve as your guide to preventive care, empowering you to make informed choices that prioritize your bone health and well-being. Together, let us embark on this journey towards stronger bones, healthier bodies, and a brighter future.

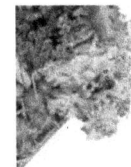

WEEKLY MEAL PLANNER

				GROCERY LIST
MONDAY	BREAKFAST			
	LUNCH			
	DINNER			
TUESDAY	BREAKFAST			
	LUNCH			
	DINNER			
WEDNESDAY	BREAKFAST			
	LUNCH			
	DINNER			
THURSDAY	BREAKFAST			
	LUNCH			
	DINNER			
FRIDAY	BREAKFAST			
	LUNCH			SNACKS
	DINNER			
SARTURDAY	BREAKFAST			
	LUNCH			
	DINNER			
SUNDAY	BREAKFAST			
	LUNCH			
	DINNER			

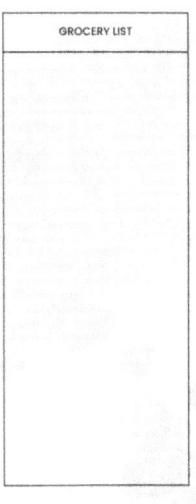

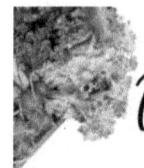

WEEKLY MEAL PLANNER

			GROCERY LIST
MONDAY	BREAKFAST		
	LUNCH		
	DINNER		
TUESDAY	BREAKFAST		
	LUNCH		
	DINNER		
WEDNESDAY	BREAKFAST		
	LUNCH		
	DINNER		
THURSDAY	BREAKFAST		
	LUNCH		
	DINNER		
FRIDAY	BREAKFAST		
	LUNCH		SNACKS
	DINNER		
SARTURDAY	BREAKFAST		
	LUNCH		
	DINNER		
SUNDAY	BREAKFAST		
	LUNCH		
	DINNER		

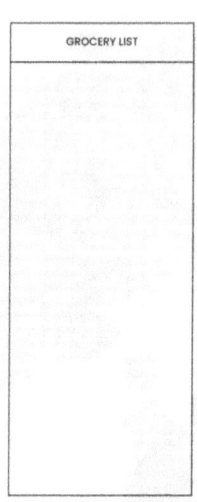

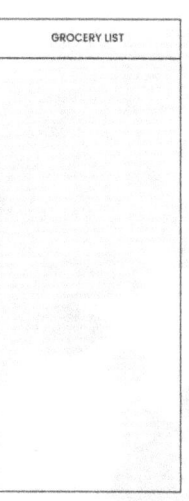

WEEKLY MEAL PLANNER

MONDAY	BREAKFAST	
	LUNCH	
	DINNER	
TUESDAY	BREAKFAST	
	LUNCH	
	DINNER	
WEDNESDAY	BREAKFAST	
	LUNCH	
	DINNER	
THURSDAY	BREAKFAST	
	LUNCH	
	DINNER	
FRIDAY	BREAKFAST	
	LUNCH	
	DINNER	
SARTURDAY	BREAKFAST	
	LUNCH	
	DINNER	
SUNDAY	BREAKFAST	
	LUNCH	
	DINNER	

GROCERY LIST

SNACKS

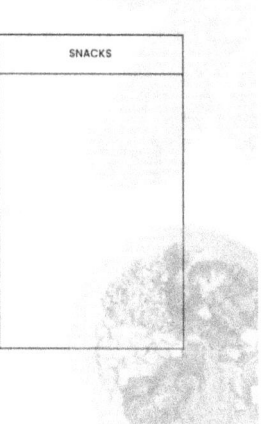

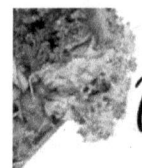

WEEKLY MEAL PLANNER

			GROCERY LIST
MONDAY	BREAKFAST		
	LUNCH		
	DINNER		
TUESDAY	BREAKFAST		
	LUNCH		
	DINNER		
WEDNESDAY	BREAKFAST		
	LUNCH		
	DINNER		
THURSDAY	BREAKFAST		
	LUNCH		
	DINNER		
FRIDAY	BREAKFAST		
	LUNCH		
	DINNER		
SARTURDAY	BREAKFAST		
	LUNCH		
	DINNER		
SUNDAY	BREAKFAST		
	LUNCH		
	DINNER		

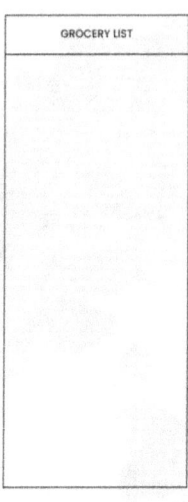

SNACKS

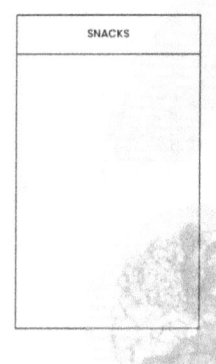

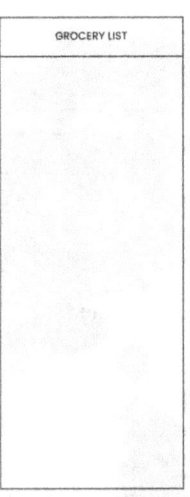

WEEKLY MEAL PLANNER

			GROCERY LIST
MONDAY	BREAKFAST		
	LUNCH		
	DINNER		
TUESDAY	BREAKFAST		
	LUNCH		
	DINNER		
WEDNESDAY	BREAKFAST		
	LUNCH		
	DINNER		
THURSDAY	BREAKFAST		
	LUNCH		
	DINNER		
FRIDAY	BREAKFAST		SNACKS
	LUNCH		
	DINNER		
SARTURDAY	BREAKFAST		
	LUNCH		
	DINNER		
SUNDAY	BREAKFAST		
	LUNCH		
	DINNER		

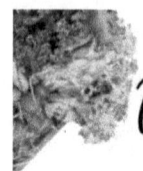

WEEKLY MEAL PLANNER

			GROCERY LIST
MONDAY	BREAKFAST		
	LUNCH		
	DINNER		
TUESDAY	BREAKFAST		
	LUNCH		
	DINNER		
WEDNESDAY	BREAKFAST		
	LUNCH		
	DINNER		
THURSDAY	BREAKFAST		
	LUNCH		
	DINNER		
FRIDAY	BREAKFAST		
	LUNCH		
	DINNER		
SARTURDAY	BREAKFAST		
	LUNCH		
	DINNER		
SUNDAY	BREAKFAST		
	LUNCH		
	DINNER		

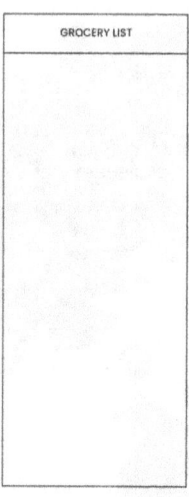

SNACKS

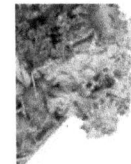

WEEKLY MEAL PLANNER

				GROCERY LIST
MONDAY	BREAKFAST			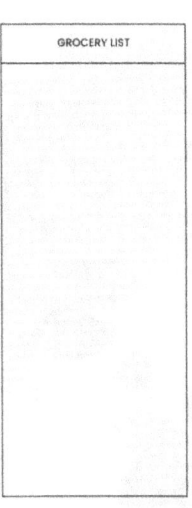
	LUNCH			
	DINNER			
TUESDAY	BREAKFAST			
	LUNCH			
	DINNER			
WEDNESDAY	BREAKFAST			
	LUNCH			
	DINNER			
THURSDAY	BREAKFAST			
	LUNCH			
	DINNER			
FRIDAY	BREAKFAST			SNACKS
	LUNCH			
	DINNER			
SARTURDAY	BREAKFAST			
	LUNCH			
	DINNER			
SUNDAY	BREAKFAST			
	LUNCH			
	DINNER			

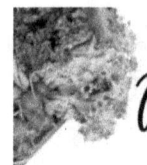

WEEKLY MEAL PLANNER

				GROCERY LIST
MONDAY	BREAKFAST			
	LUNCH			
	DINNER			
TUESDAY	BREAKFAST			
	LUNCH			
	DINNER			
WEDNESDAY	BREAKFAST			
	LUNCH			
	DINNER			
THURSDAY	BREAKFAST			
	LUNCH			
	DINNER			
FRIDAY	BREAKFAST			
	LUNCH			SNACKS
	DINNER			
SARTURDAY	BREAKFAST			
	LUNCH			
	DINNER			
SUNDAY	BREAKFAST			
	LUNCH			
	DINNER			

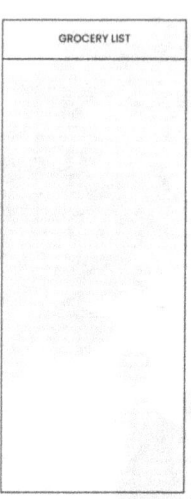
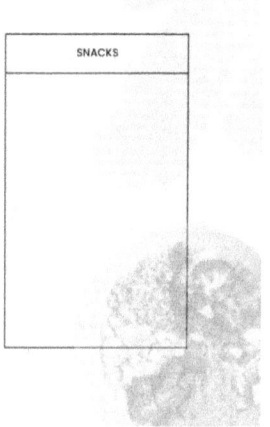

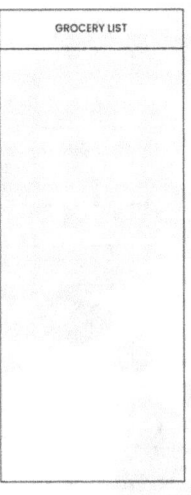

WEEKLY MEAL PLANNER

				GROCERY LIST
MONDAY	BREAKFAST			
	LUNCH			
	DINNER			
TUESDAY	BREAKFAST			
	LUNCH			
	DINNER			
WEDNESDAY	BREAKFAST			
	LUNCH			
	DINNER			
THURSDAY	BREAKFAST			
	LUNCH			
	DINNER			
FRIDAY	BREAKFAST			SNACKS
	LUNCH			
	DINNER			
SARTURDAY	BREAKFAST			
	LUNCH			
	DINNER			
SUNDAY	BREAKFAST			
	LUNCH			
	DINNER			

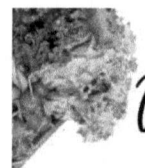

WEEKLY MEAL PLANNER

MONDAY	BREAKFAST		
	LUNCH		
	DINNER		
TUESDAY	BREAKFAST		
	LUNCH		
	DINNER		
WEDNESDAY	BREAKFAST		
	LUNCH		
	DINNER		
THURSDAY	BREAKFAST		
	LUNCH		
	DINNER		
FRIDAY	BREAKFAST		
	LUNCH		
	DINNER		
SARTURDAY	BREAKFAST		
	LUNCH		
	DINNER		
SUNDAY	BREAKFAST		
	LUNCH		
	DINNER		

GROCERY LIST

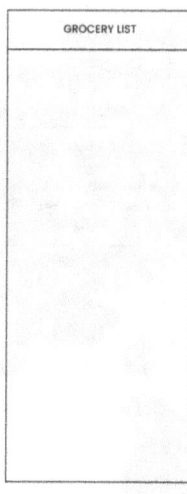

SNACKS

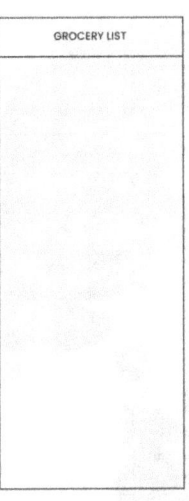

WEEKLY MEAL PLANNER

MONDAY	BREAKFAST	
	LUNCH	
	DINNER	
TUESDAY	BREAKFAST	
	LUNCH	
	DINNER	
WEDNESDAY	BREAKFAST	
	LUNCH	
	DINNER	
THURSDAY	BREAKFAST	
	LUNCH	
	DINNER	
FRIDAY	BREAKFAST	
	LUNCH	
	DINNER	
SARTURDAY	BREAKFAST	
	LUNCH	
	DINNER	
SUNDAY	BREAKFAST	
	LUNCH	
	DINNER	

GROCERY LIST

SNACKS

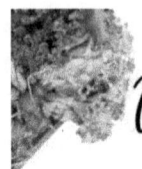

WEEKLY MEAL PLANNER

			GROCERY LIST
MONDAY	BREAKFAST		
	LUNCH		
	DINNER		
TUESDAY	BREAKFAST		
	LUNCH		
	DINNER		
WEDNESDAY	BREAKFAST		
	LUNCH		
	DINNER		
THURSDAY	BREAKFAST		
	LUNCH		
	DINNER		
FRIDAY	BREAKFAST		SNACKS
	LUNCH		
	DINNER		
SARTURDAY	BREAKFAST		
	LUNCH		
	DINNER		
SUNDAY	BREAKFAST		
	LUNCH		
	DINNER		

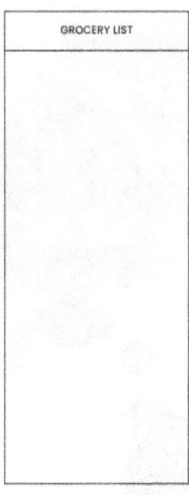

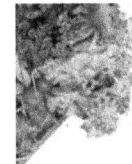

WEEKLY MEAL PLANNER

MONDAY	BREAKFAST	
	LUNCH	
	DINNER	
TUESDAY	BREAKFAST	
	LUNCH	
	DINNER	
WEDNESDAY	BREAKFAST	
	LUNCH	
	DINNER	
THURSDAY	BREAKFAST	
	LUNCH	
	DINNER	
FRIDAY	BREAKFAST	
	LUNCH	
	DINNER	
SARTURDAY	BREAKFAST	
	LUNCH	
	DINNER	
SUNDAY	BREAKFAST	
	LUNCH	
	DINNER	

GROCERY LIST

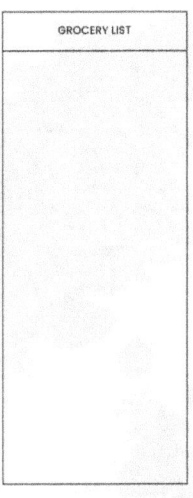

SNACKS

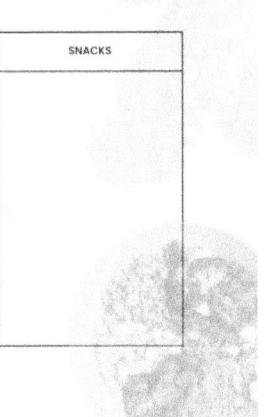

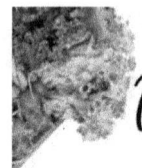

WEEKLY MEAL PLANNER

				GROCERY LIST
MONDAY	BREAKFAST			
	LUNCH			
	DINNER			
TUESDAY	BREAKFAST			
	LUNCH			
	DINNER			
WEDNESDAY	BREAKFAST			
	LUNCH			
	DINNER			
THURSDAY	BREAKFAST			
	LUNCH			
	DINNER			
FRIDAY	BREAKFAST			
	LUNCH			SNACKS
	DINNER			
SARTURDAY	BREAKFAST			
	LUNCH			
	DINNER			
SUNDAY	BREAKFAST			
	LUNCH			
	DINNER			

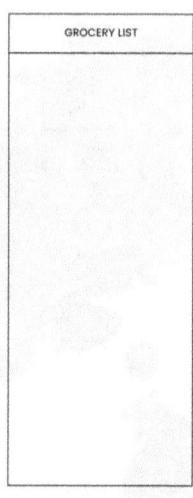

www.ingramcontent.com/pod-product-compliance
Lightning Source LLC
Chambersburg PA
CBHW070958290526
45795CB00005B/1692